LIGHT

Andrew Woodhead

Illustrated by Alan Chen

ISBN 978-0-6487112-2-3

thefinchfoundation.com

How to contact the Author?

To ask a question about the book, contact the author, or report a mistake in the text, please write to Andrew Woodhead, at; caring@designtobias.com

This book has been produced in partnership with Design Tobias, a Human-centred design consultancy based in Sydney.

We are driven by impact, not profits. All money raised from the sale of this book will be spent on improving Mental Health Services in Australia.

MEMORIES

This book is dedicated to and in loving memory of:

The Grandma I sadly never knew - Mavis

Robert John Townsend

Chester Charles Bennington

ACKNOWLEDGEMENTS

There are so many people who have helped me on the road to recovery, and the creation of this book.

First and foremost, I want to thank my sister Sarah, who has been my rock through many a dark day. I couldn't have done it without you.

To Tara, my psychologist, who always greeted me with a warming smile and who continues to support me with the challenges I face. To my Tobias family who were the best and most supportive team I could ever have wished for. To the Directors that have backed and helped me drive this project forward, to Alan who has created these magnificent illustrations and to Braddon who has brought it all together and exercised immense patience!

Lastly a huge thank you to you, if you've bought this book. If this book helps just one person then that's a result, but the more we can collectively help the better...our mission continues!

PREFACE

Before you begin, I want you to know that I have suffered from anxiety and depression and in my darkest hour I considered taking my life. I chose not to, but as part of my recovery I am compelled to try and help those suffering. Whether you or a loved one is struggling with the stresses and strains of everyday life, or if there is an overwhelming feeling that the burden is just too much, it's important to know that you are not alone and that there is help out there.

This book contains tips and tricks that myself and many others have found helpful in managing and overcoming anxiety and depression. Seeking help and support from family, friends and medical professionals is vital, but so to is trying, learning and practicing new approaches and techniques.

Everyone is on a journey through life, navigating through all the highs and the lows that come with it. Sometimes without foresight or control over what happens. During difficult periods it's necessary to use the people and the tools that can make your life that little bit easier. Throughout this book are a list of recommended activities, strategies and resources that I found helpful on my road to recovery. Some will work for you, others might not but it's a start. Lastly, please be patient and kind to yourself. If you can't, or if you find it hard, then do your best to learn. You can do this.

A.R. Woodhead

Andrew R. Woodhead

IN THE BEGINNING...

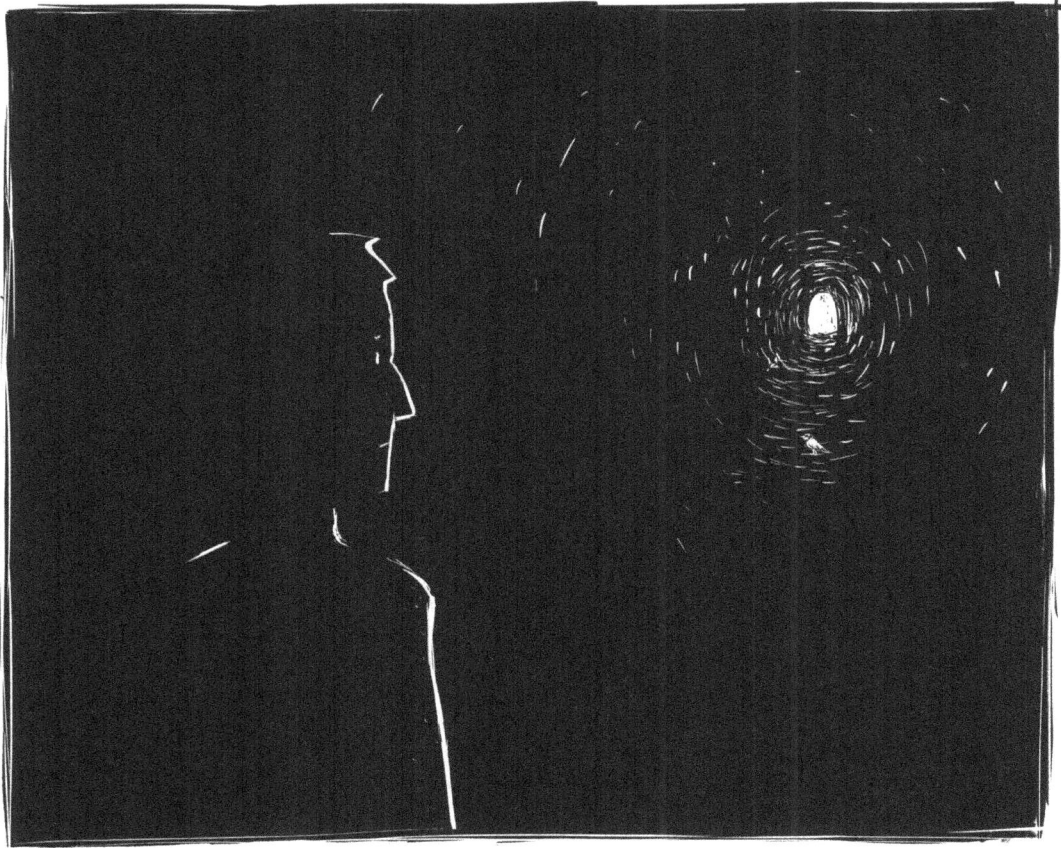

DARK

You may not feel like it right now, but there is
light at the end of the tunnel.

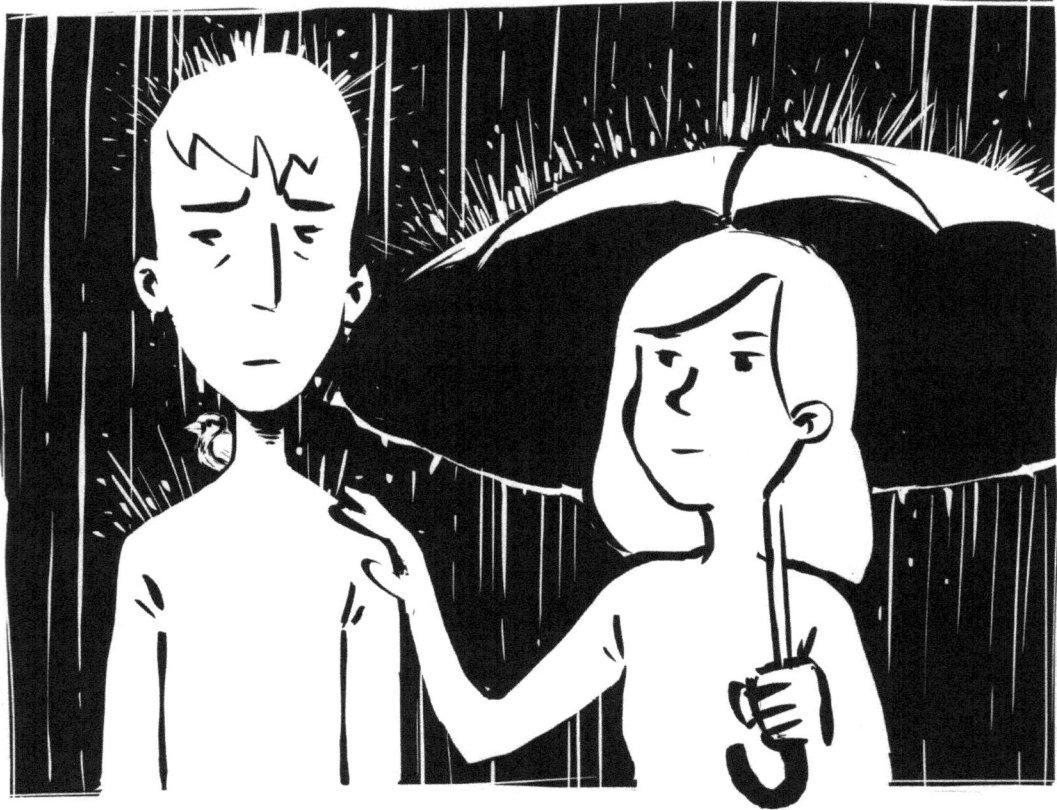

OK

It's OK, not to be OK. Recognising that is the first step. You can get through difficult times.

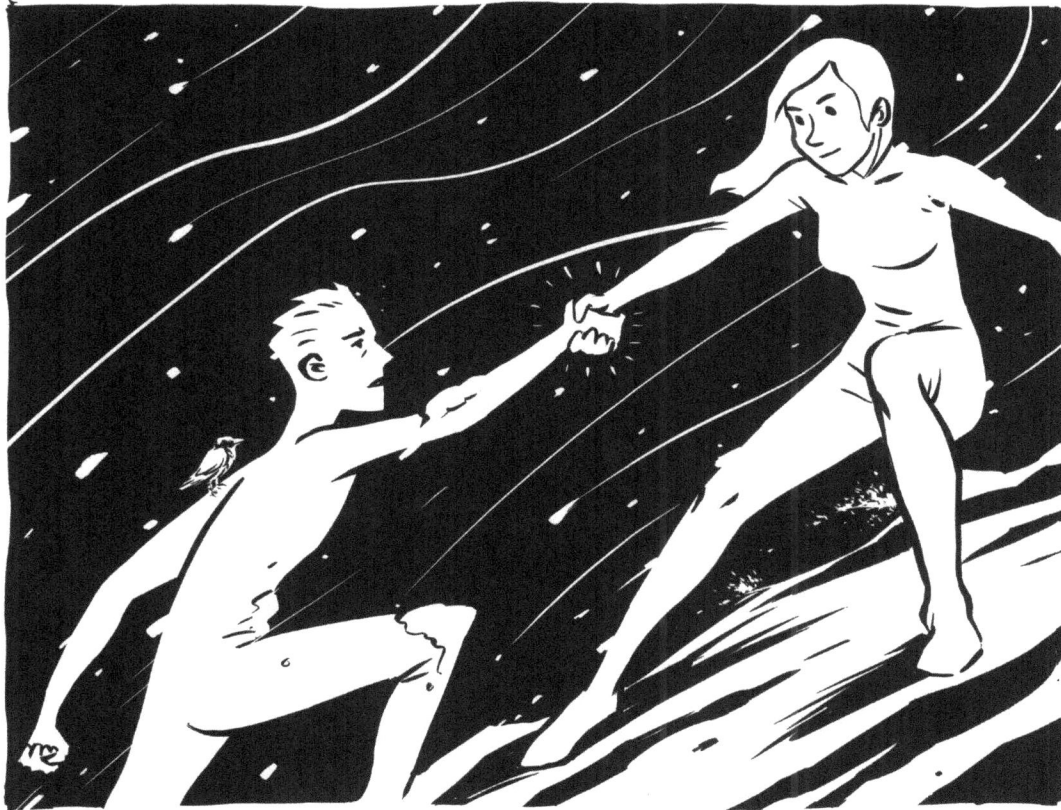

HELP

Asking for support from friends, family or professionals
is a good first step. It's important to share how you are
thinking and feeling.

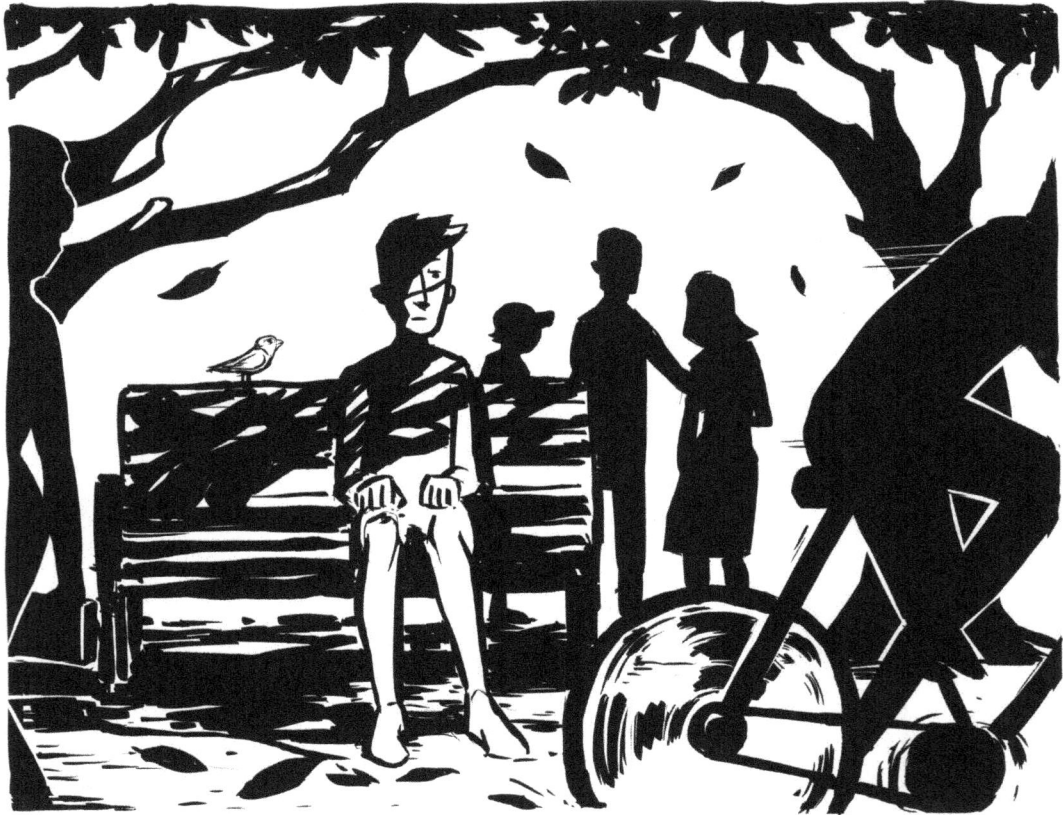

ALONE

You may feel alone, but there are people that can and will help you. Make sure you leave the house to see the people that surround you.

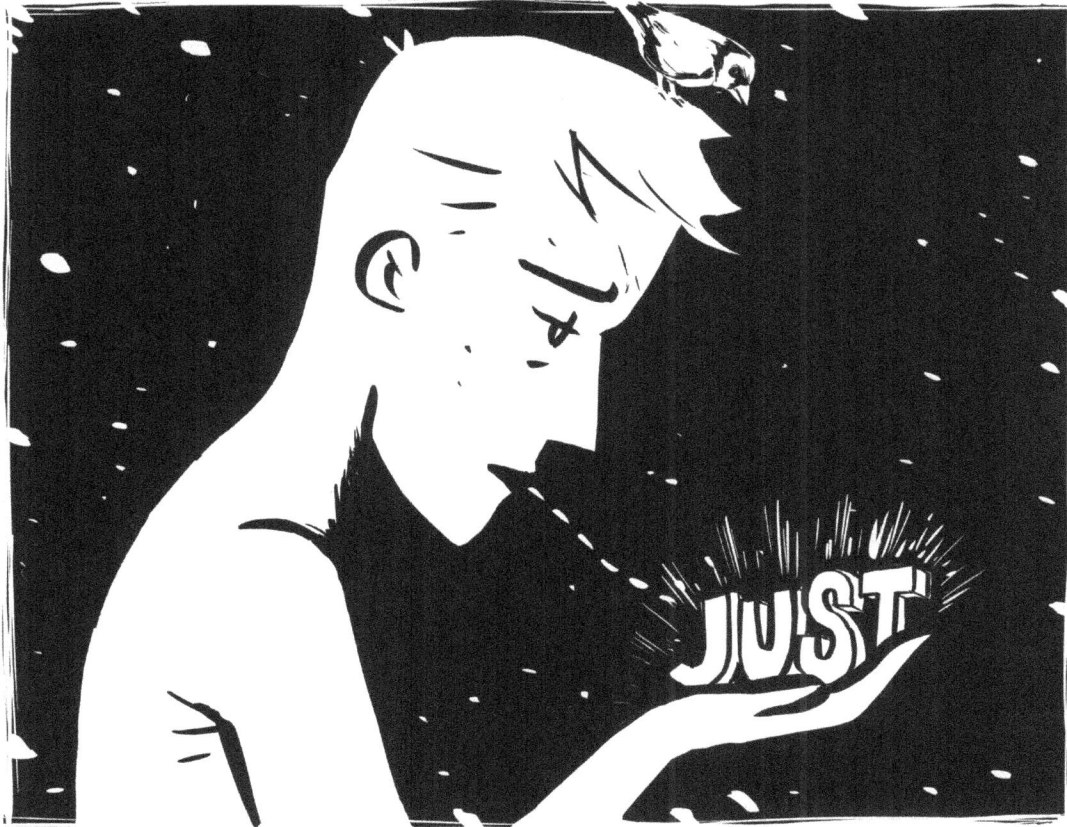

TALK

You may not feel like talking, but a problem shared is a problem halved. Open up to someone you are willing to trust, it's good to talk.

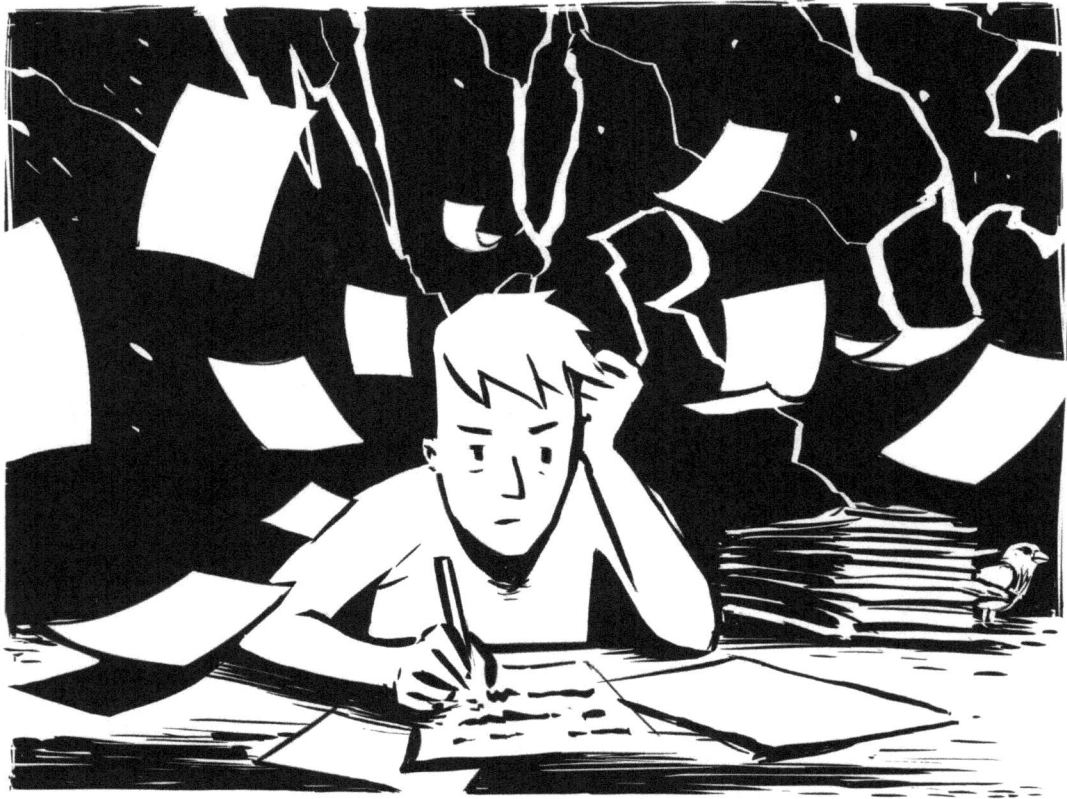

WRITE

If you don't feel like talking, that's ok. Write down anything that is causing stress, pain or upset.

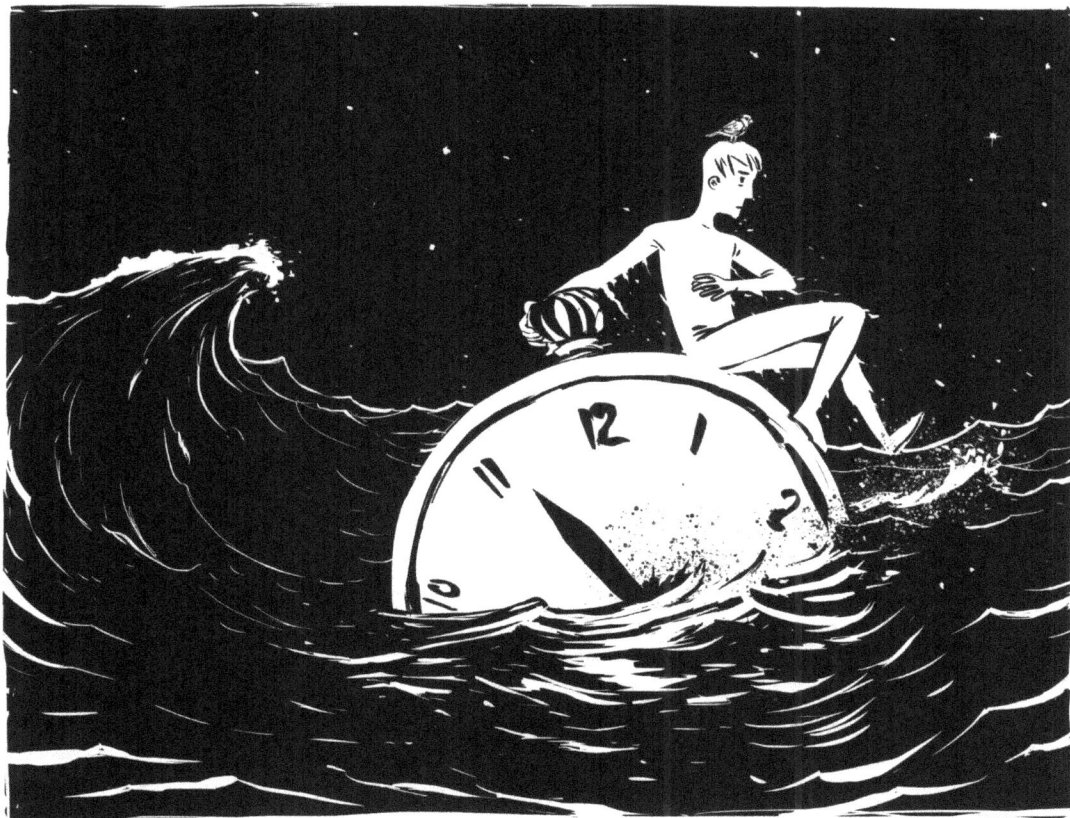

TIME

At times waves of anxiety and despair will hit you but ride the wave. Be patient and kind to yourself. The waves will get smaller.

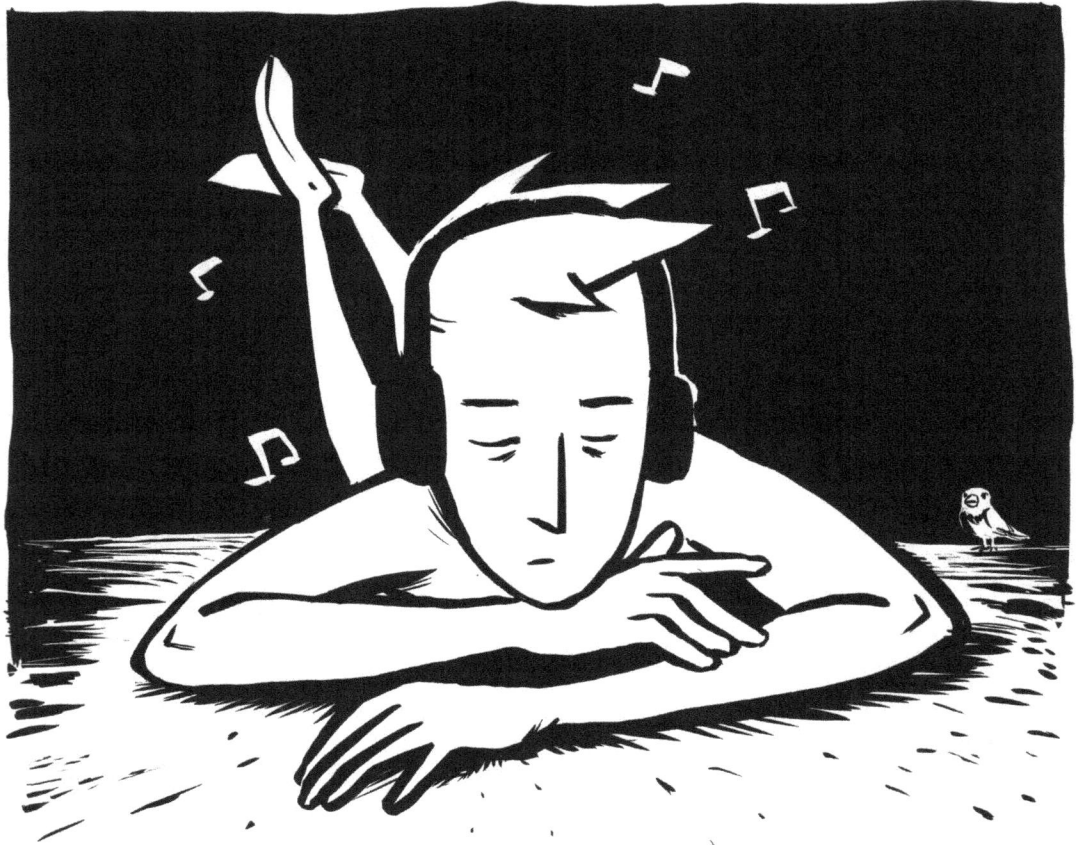

RELAX

Make time to give back to your body and mind. There are many ways to do this. Find what works for you.

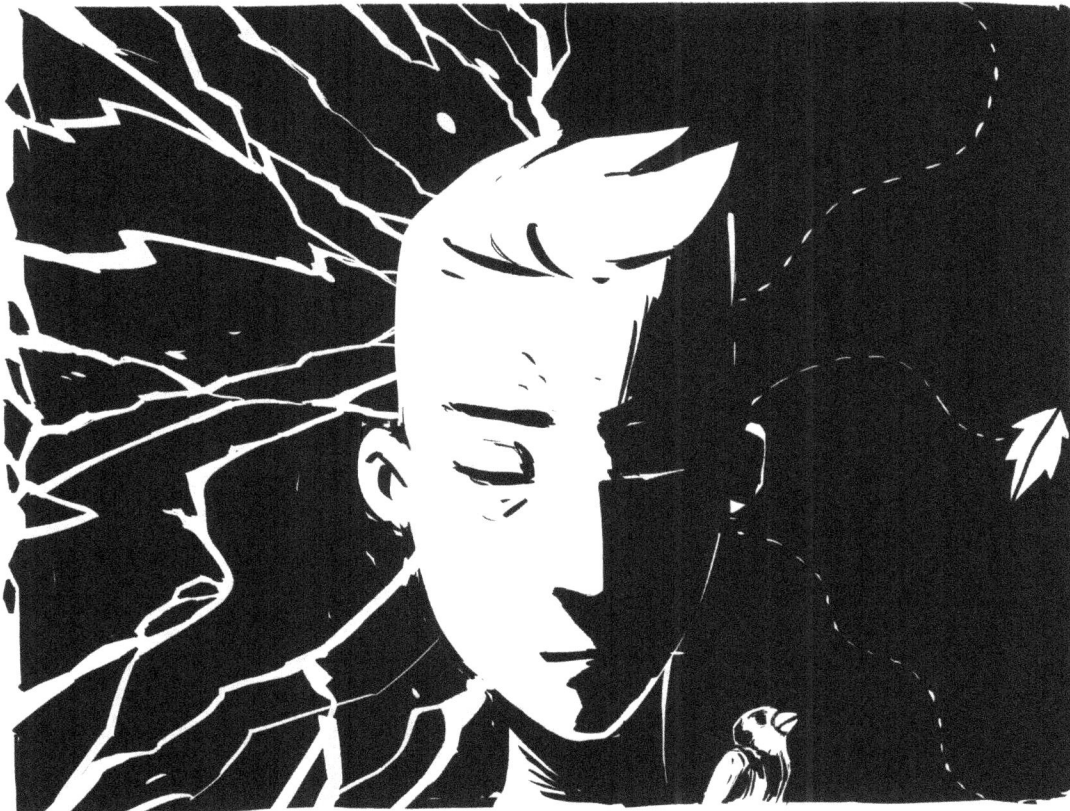

MEDITATE

Give your brain a break from the stresses and strains of life. Close your eyes and focus on your breathing. Create a happy place in your mind.

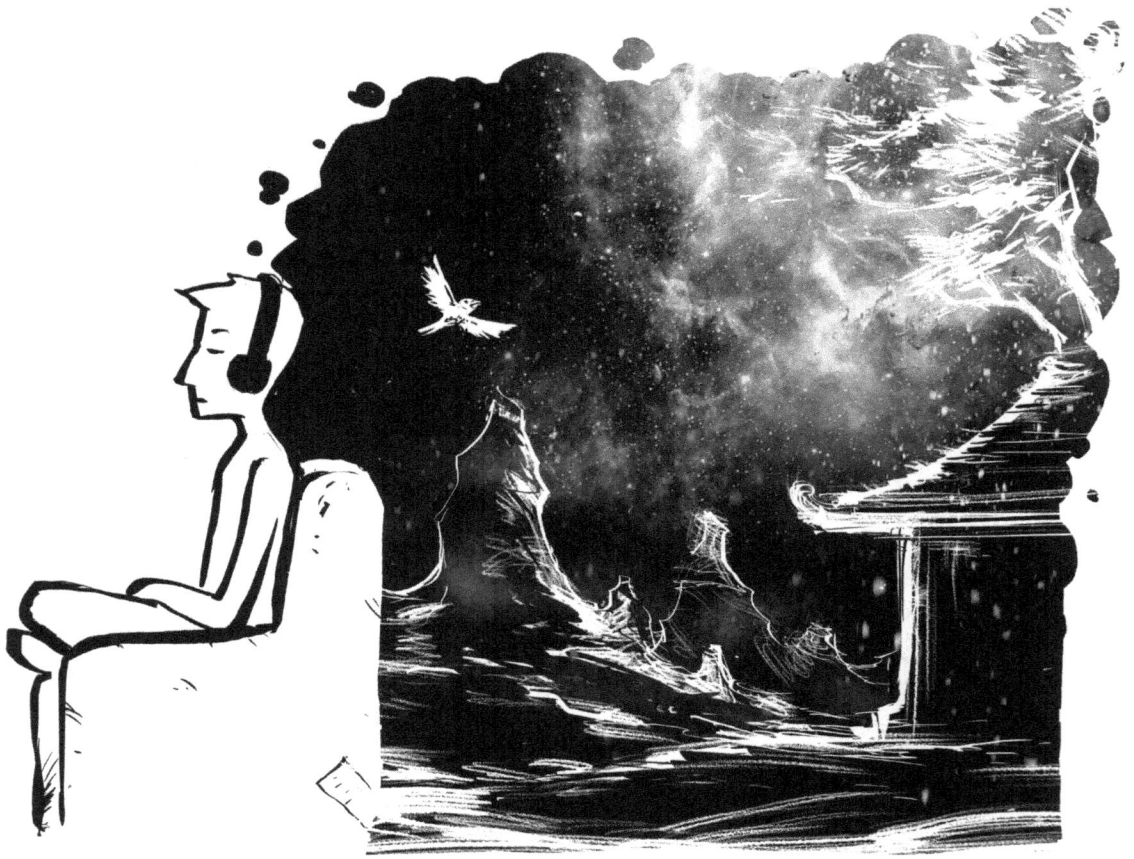

SANCTUARY

Where is your safe and happy place? Imagine what it looks and sounds like. If your mind drifts that's ok, acknowledge your thoughts and refocus.

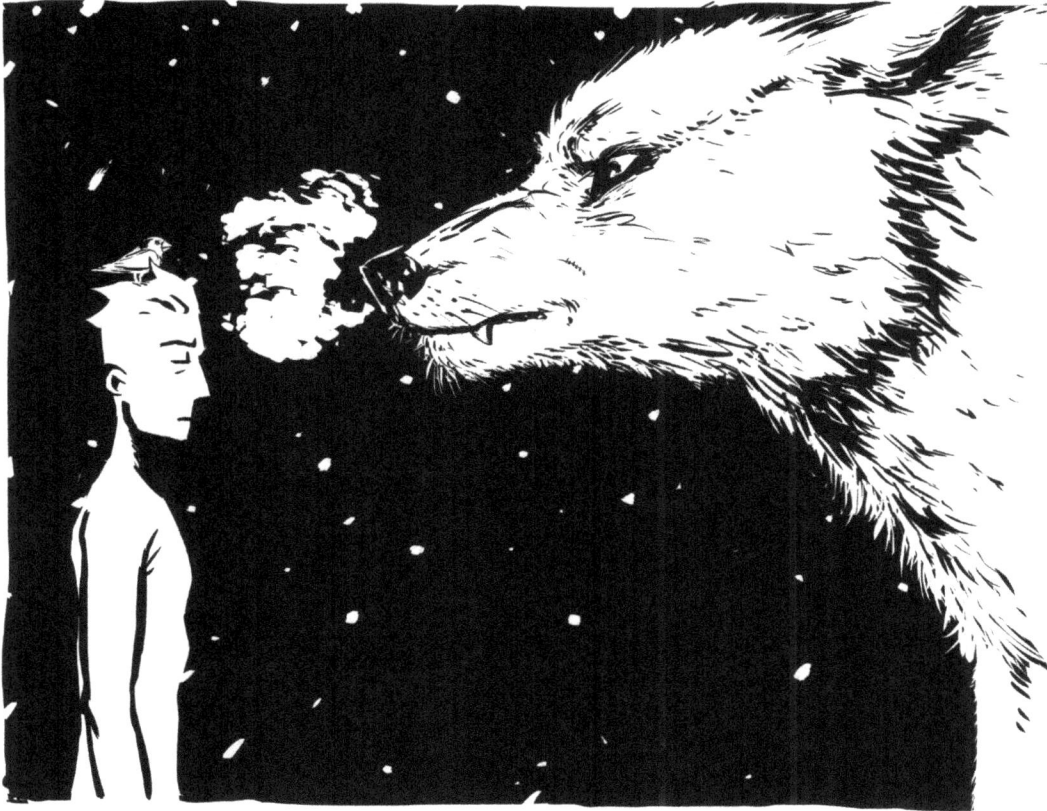

THOUGHTS

We all have different perspectives and thoughts. Some are happy, some aren't. That's normal. Do your best to accept your thoughts non judgmentally.

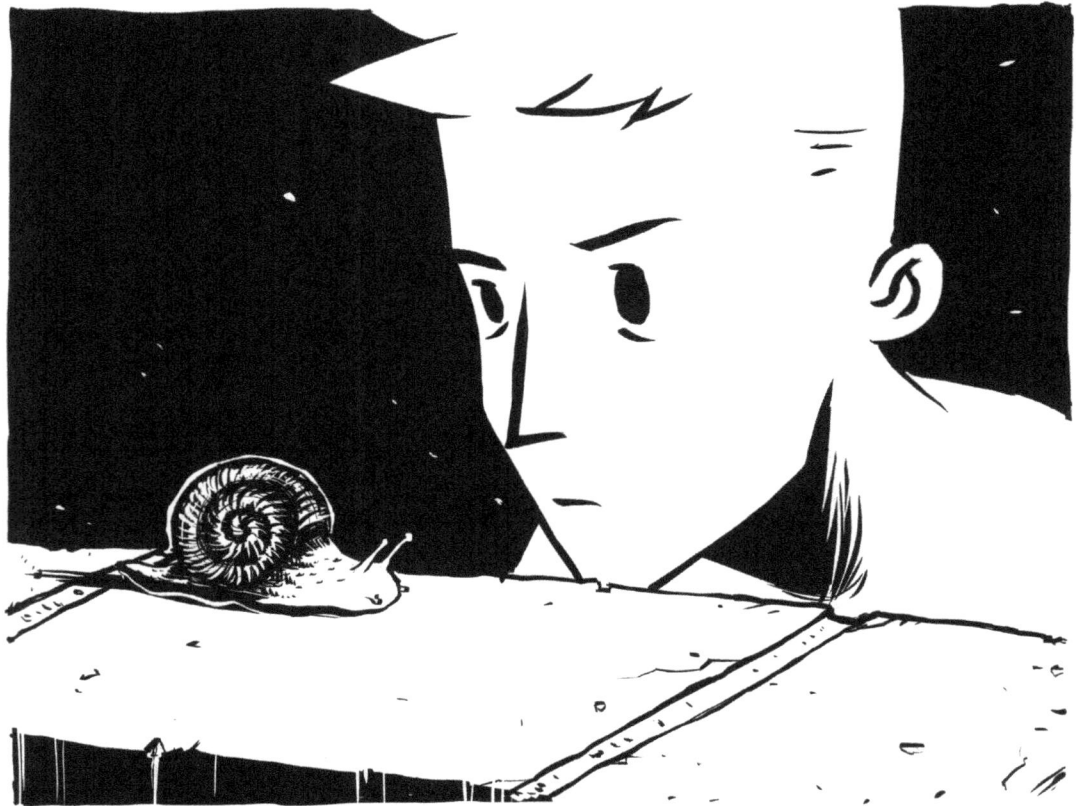

MINDFUL

Mindfulness focuses our awareness on the present moment, calmly acknowledging and accepting our feelings and thoughts. Try it. Practice it. Learn it.

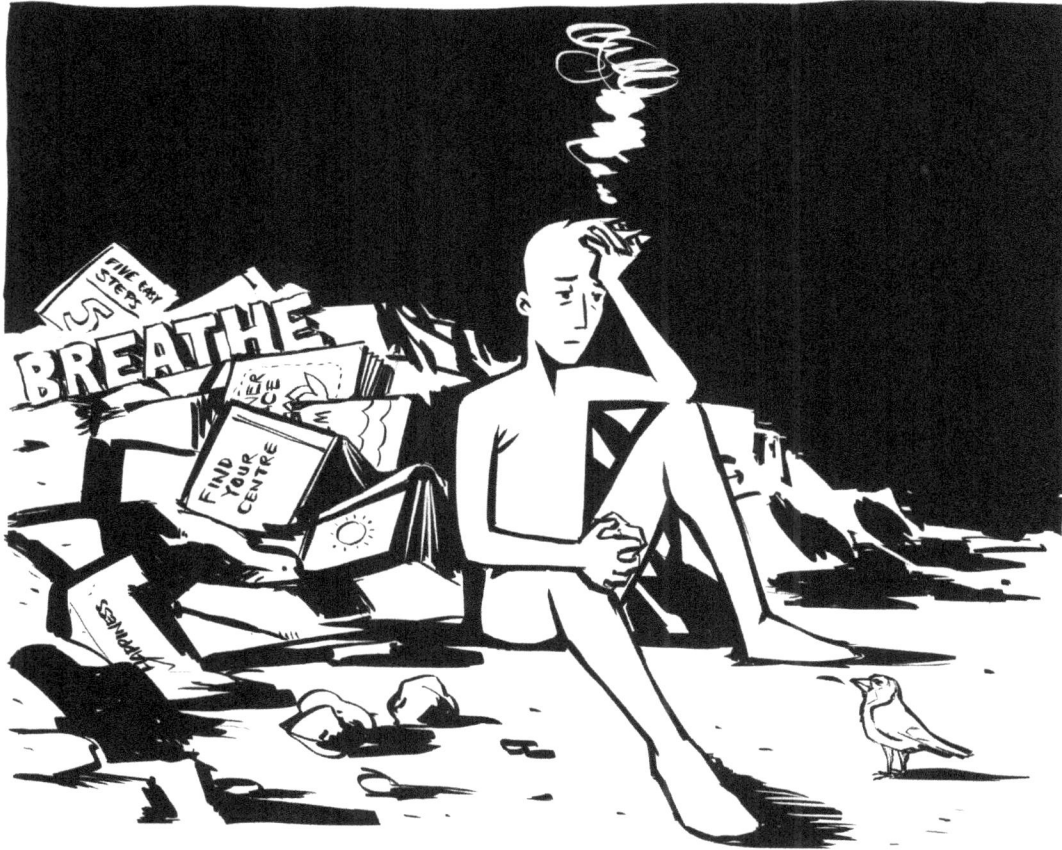

FRUSTRATION

Trying new approaches may bring frustrations. You may feel like you aren't winning but be patient, in time you will. Practice mindfulness and meditation.

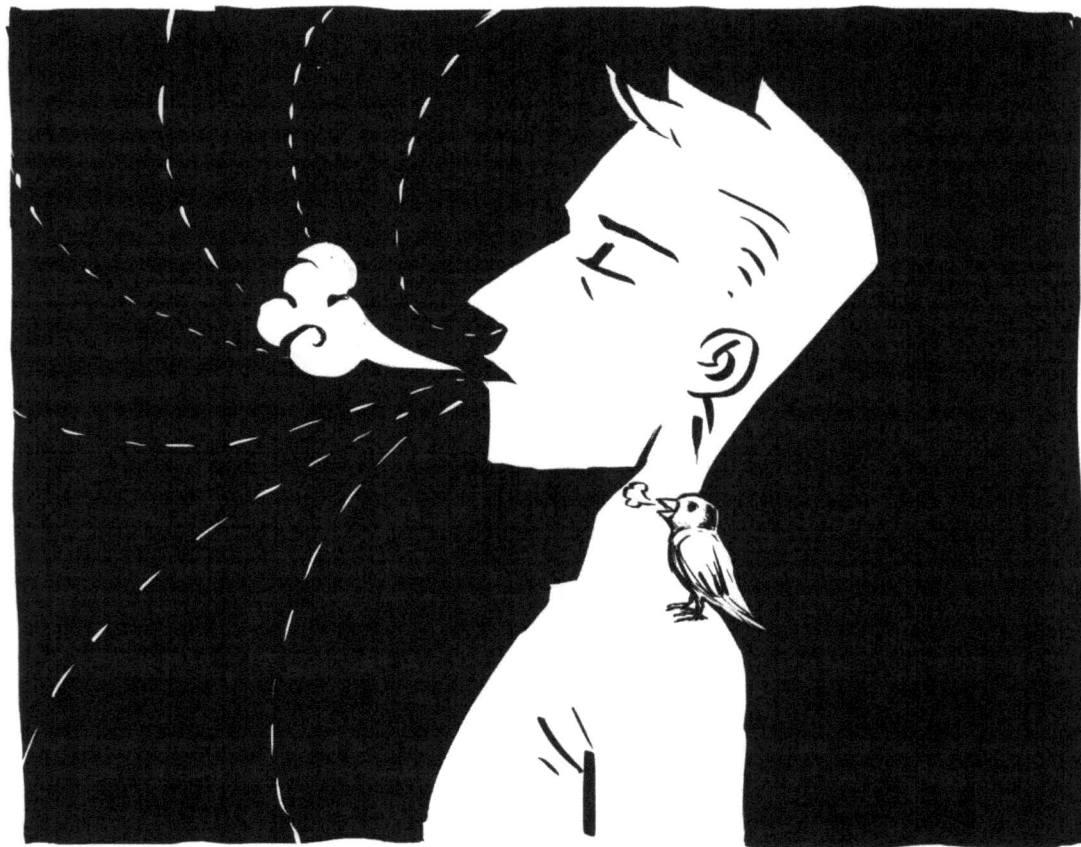

BREATHE

Breathe in deeply and exhale fully. Deep, slow breathing will help relax your body and mind. Deep breathing is a great way to respond to anxious thoughts.

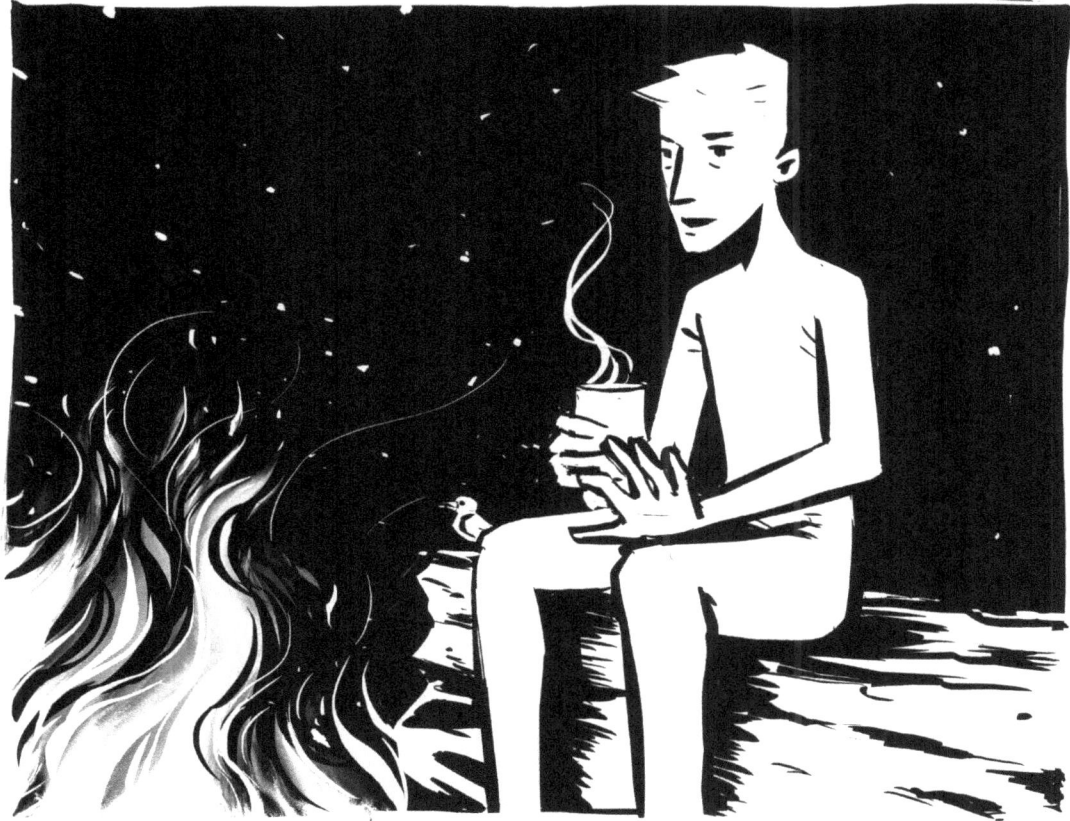

SENSES

Each day, stop for a few moments and engage with your senses. Notice unique objects around you. Touch them. Feel them. Connect with them.

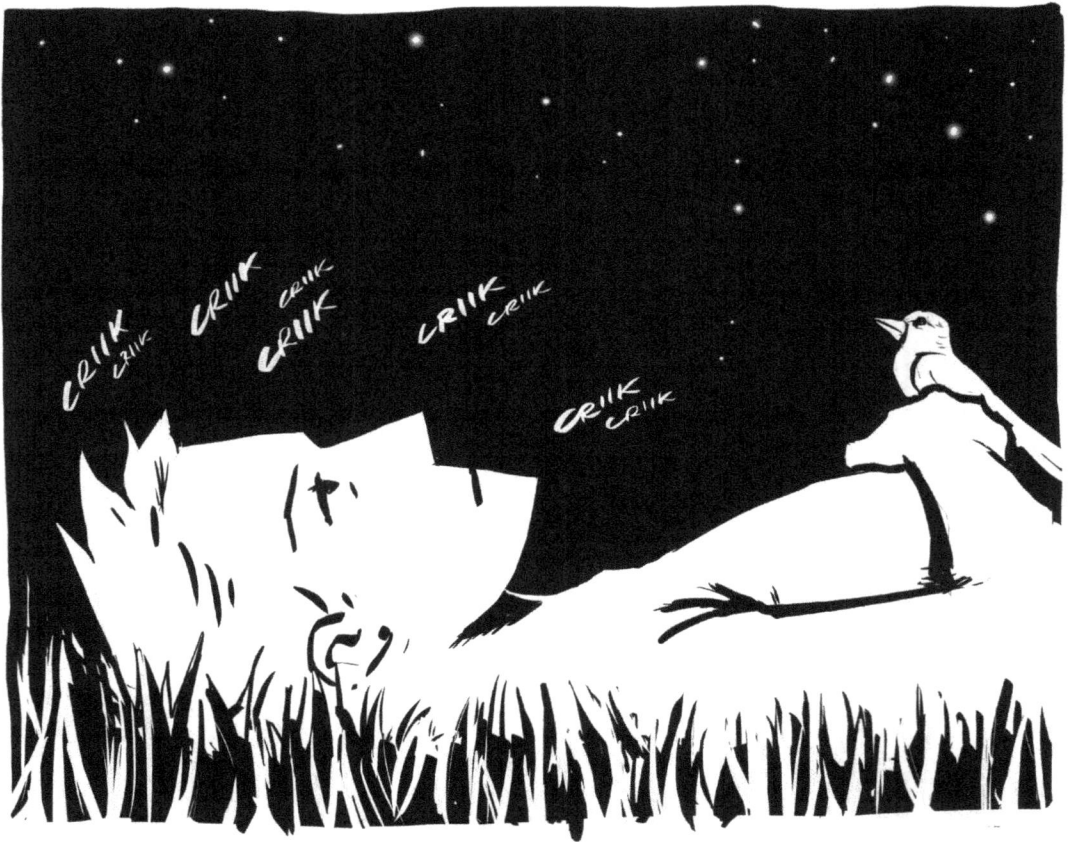

LISTEN

If life feels too hectic and noisy, go to a quiet place. Sit or lie down and enjoy the silence and tranquillity.

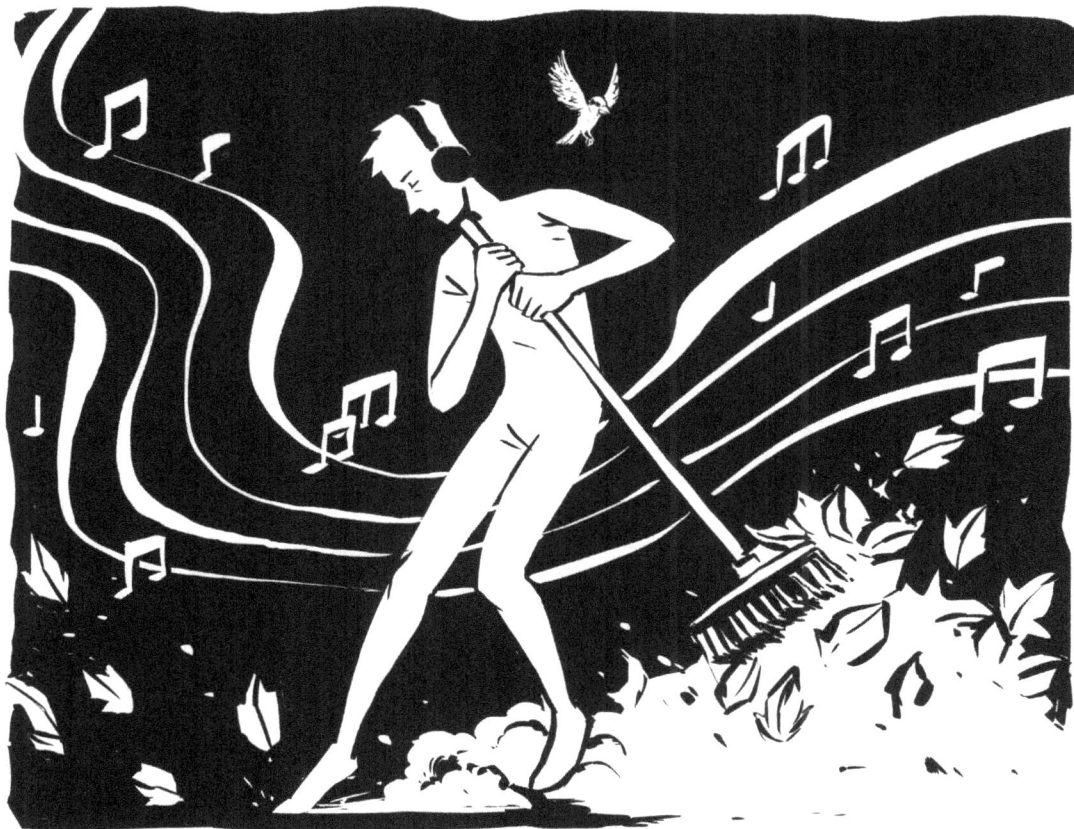

MUSIC

Put on your favourite music, have a dance and move to the beat. Get singing or playing your favourite instrument.

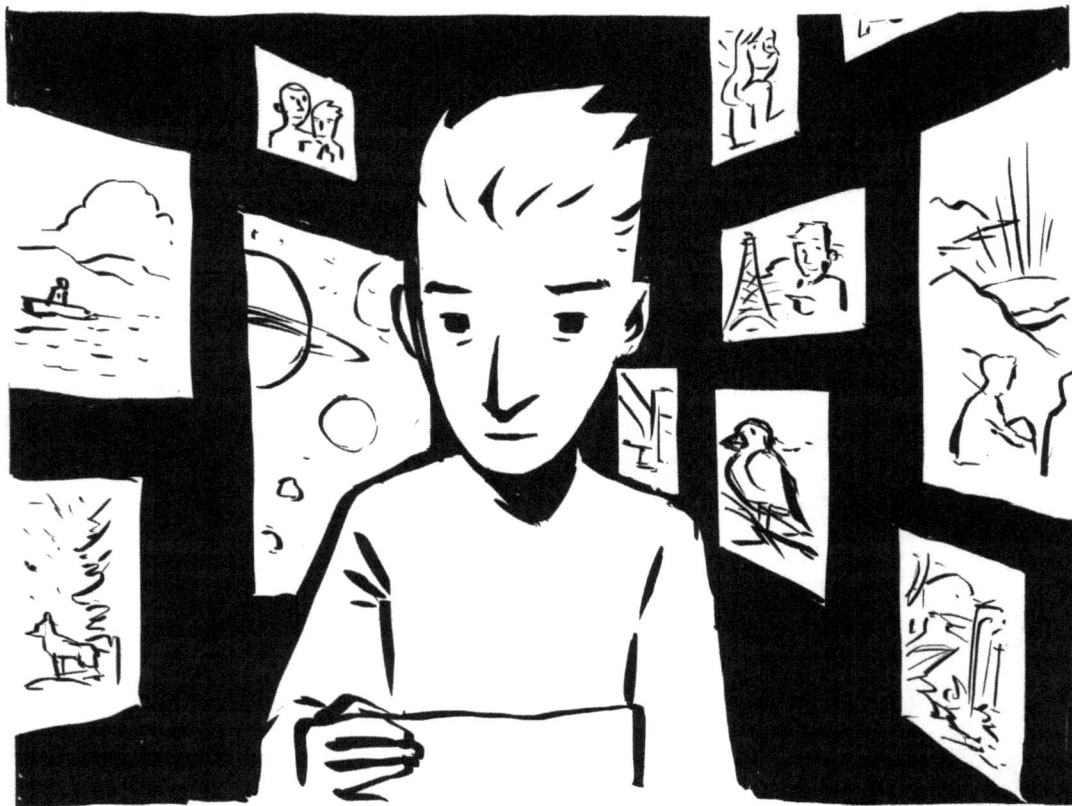

PICTURES

Observe the beauty of nature that surrounds you.
Take photos. This will help you to be present
and gain an alternative perspective.

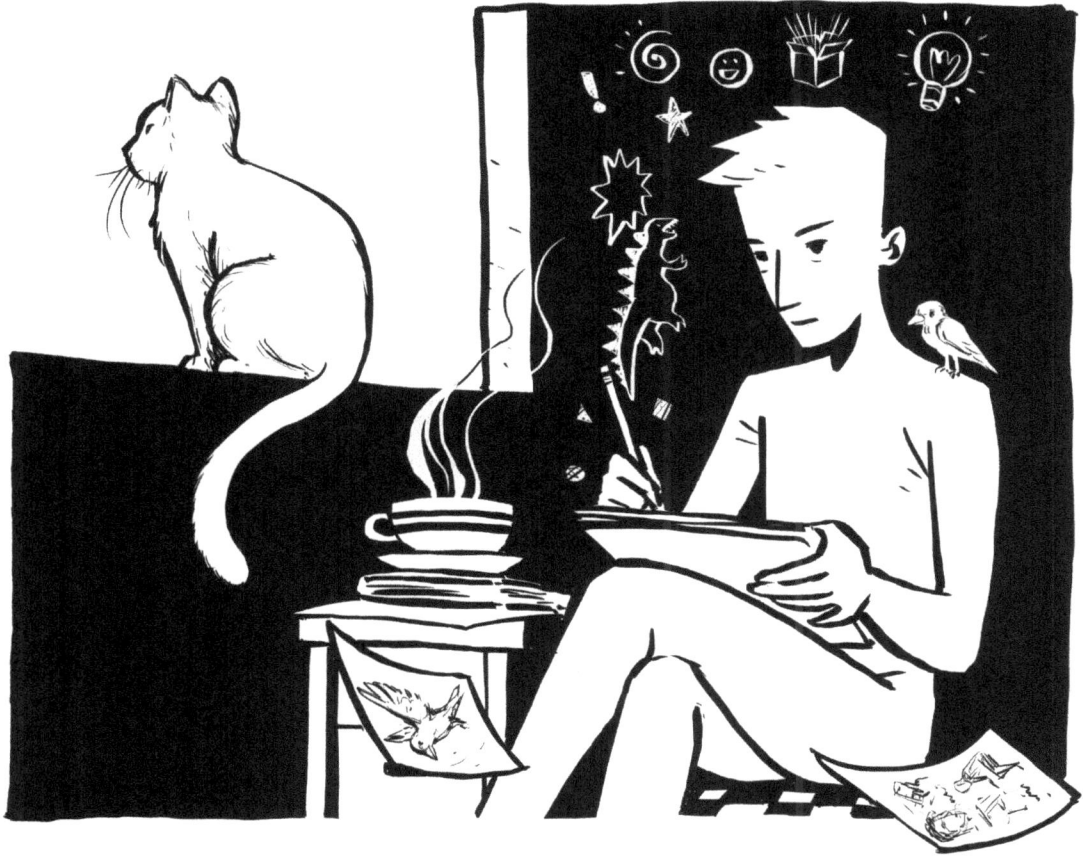

DRAW

Get out in nature and sketch. It's a therapeutic activity that can help you to relax. Experiment with it. Try it and see if it helps you.

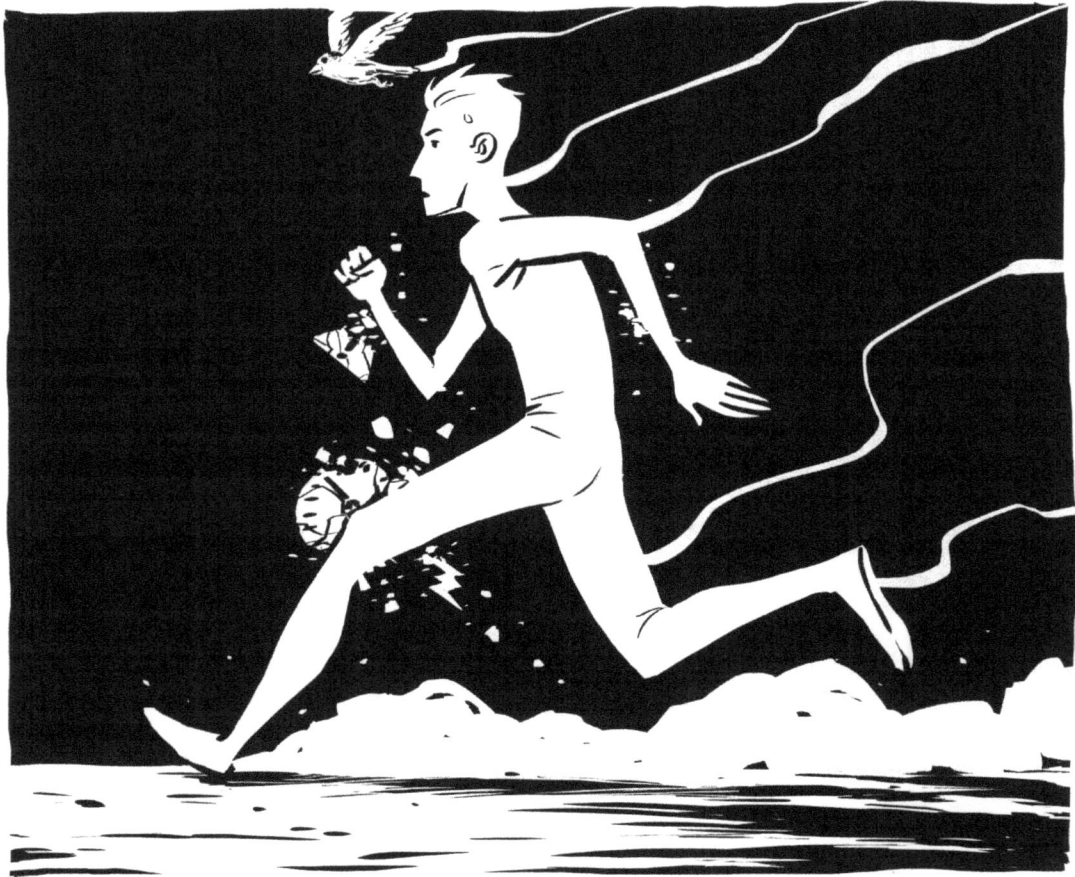

EXERCISE

Get the blood pumping around your body. Go for a walk, run or swim. It will help by releasing happy chemicals in your brain.

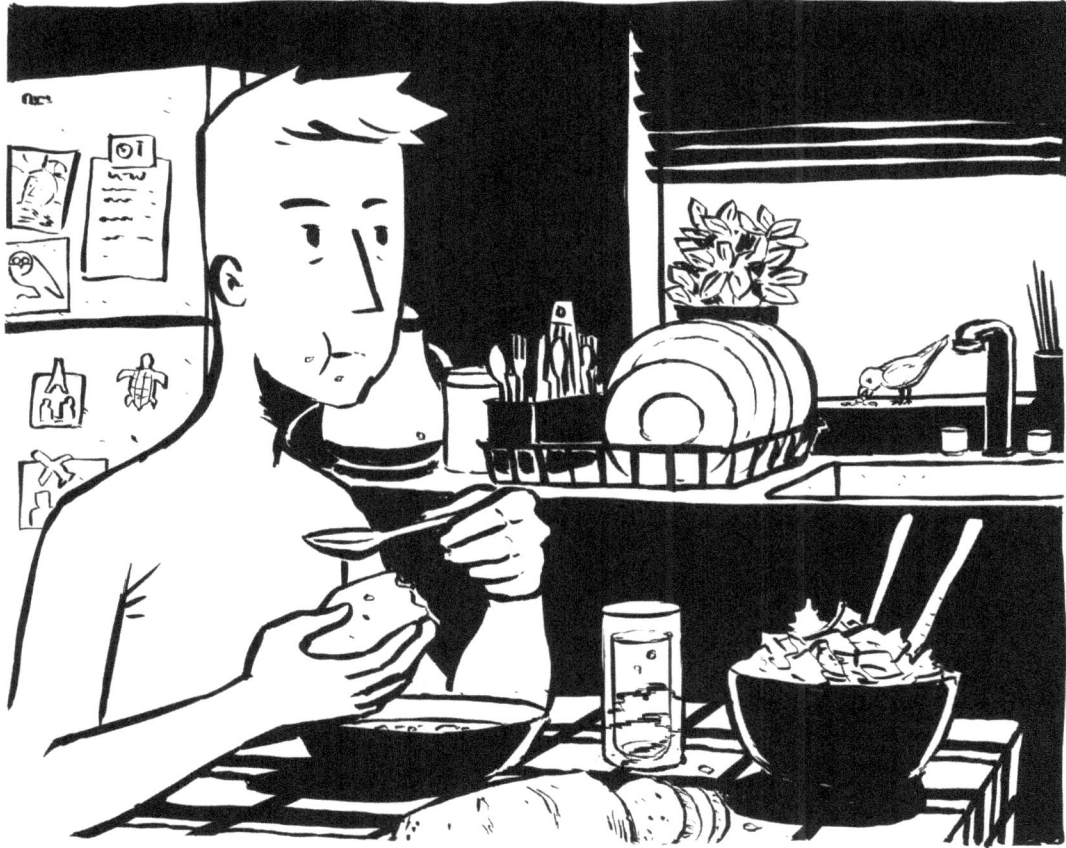

FOOD

Food is the fuel that feeds your body. You must eat, even if you don't feel like it. Focus your senses by noticing the delicious flavours in each meal.

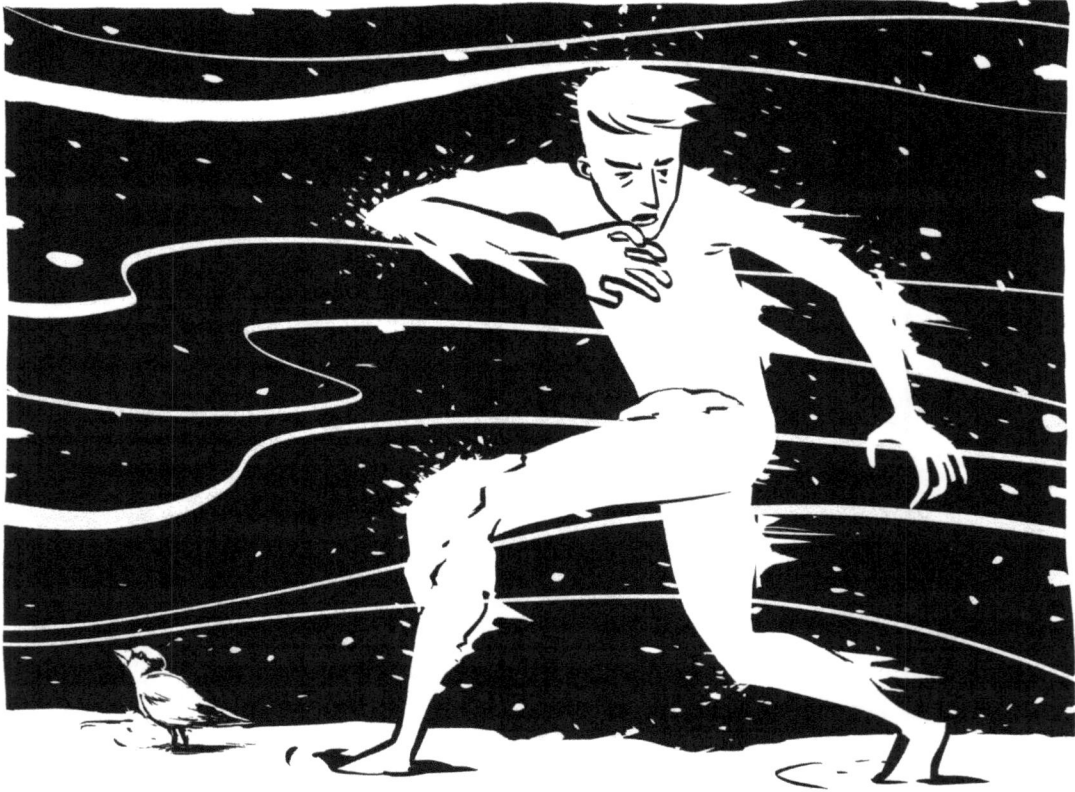

TOUGH

At times life feels tough. It can feel like it isn't getting better, or easier. But you must be patient. Time is a great healer.

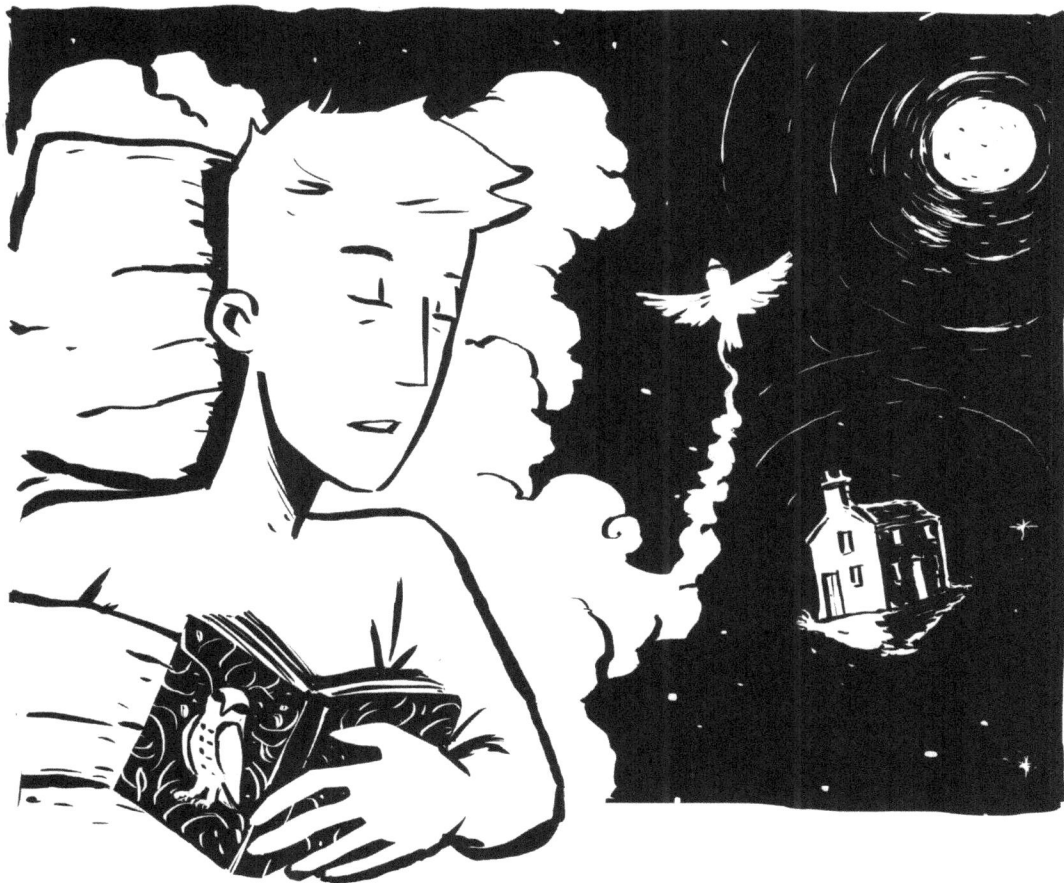

SLEEP

When life is tough, your sleep can suffer. Detach from technology and develop a routine that calms you before sleep. Use meditation or read a book.

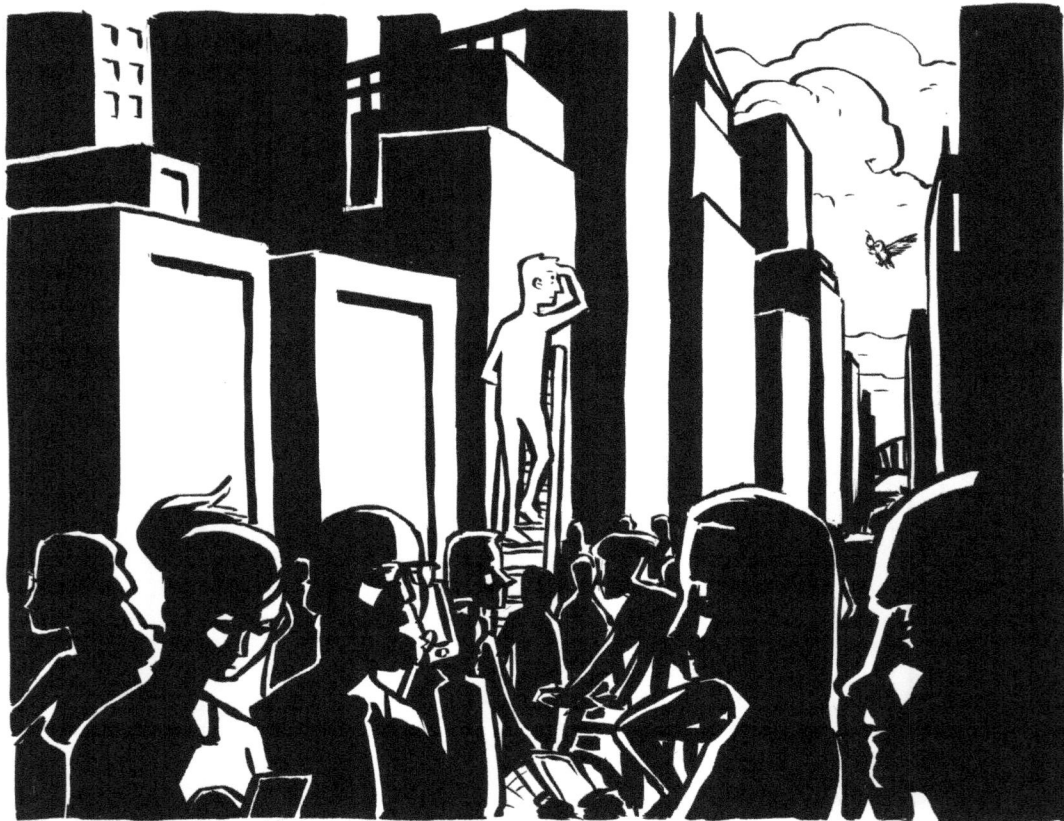

PERSPECTIVE

When we are down, we can get things out of proportion. Talk to someone you trust, share your worries and find a different perspective.

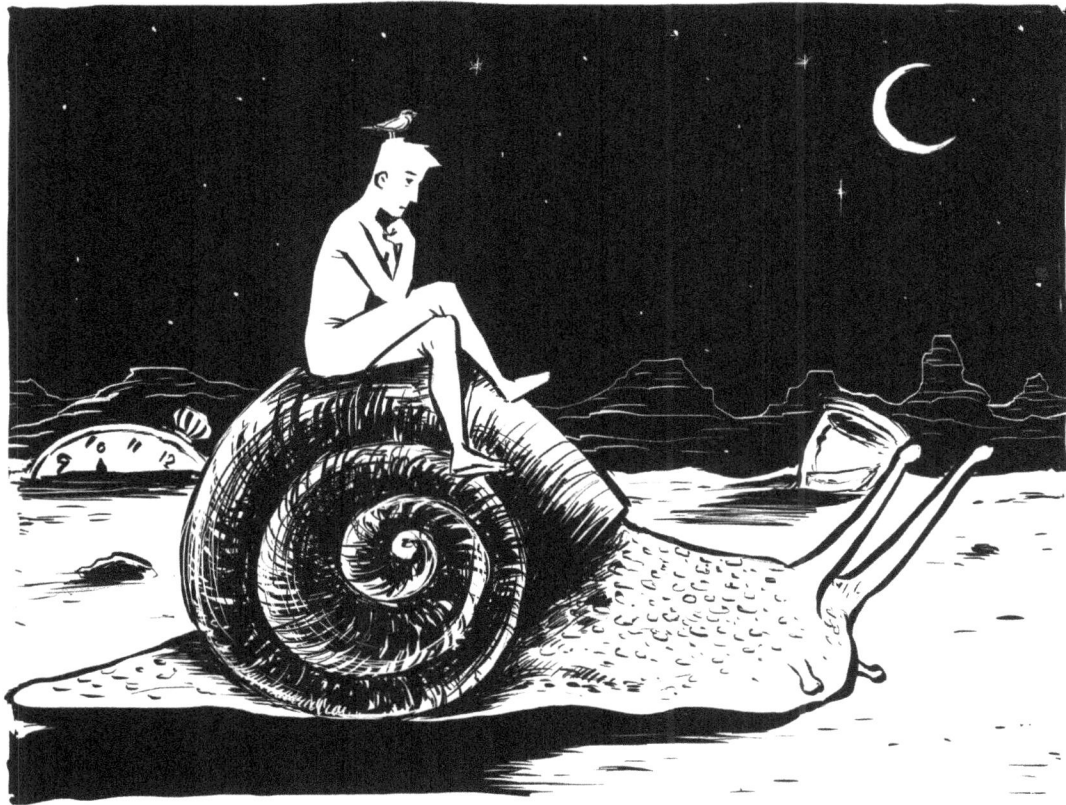

PATIENCE

Sadly, there is no quick fix but use this book and the people around you. Be patient and you will turn the corner.

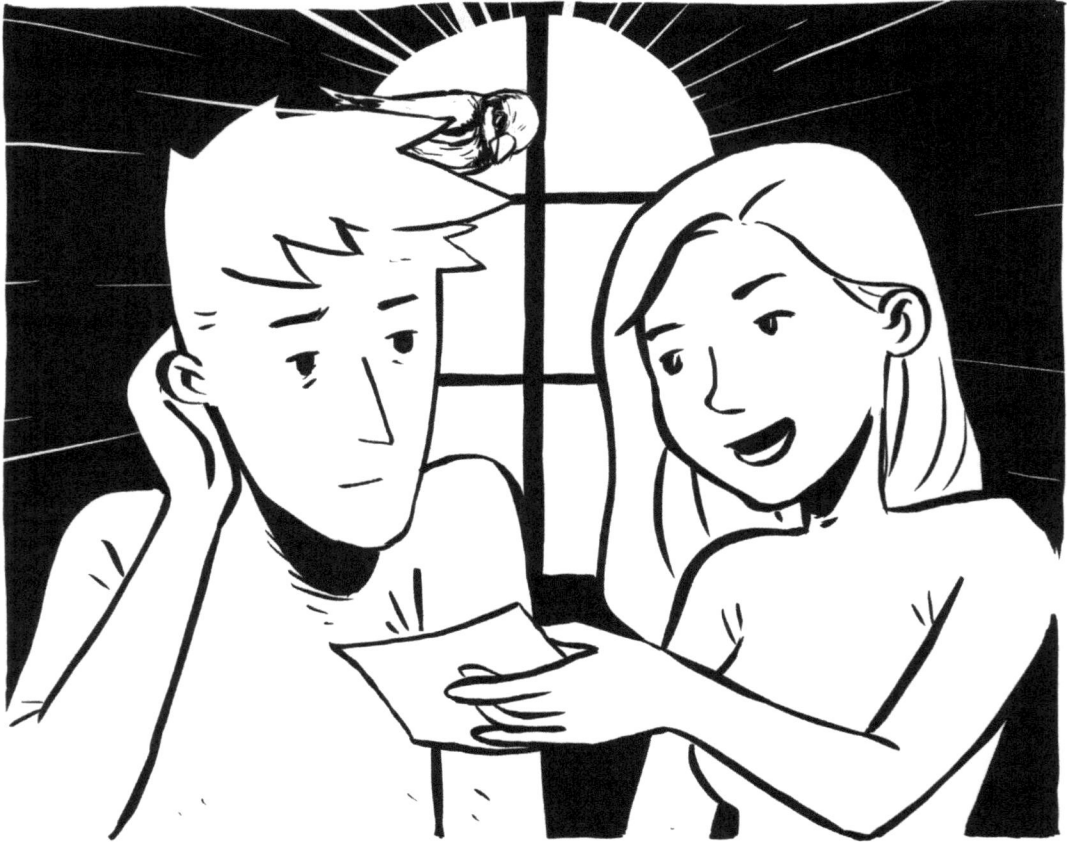

KIND

Be your own best friend. You have many qualities and if you don't believe it, then ask a close friend for 3 things that they value about you.

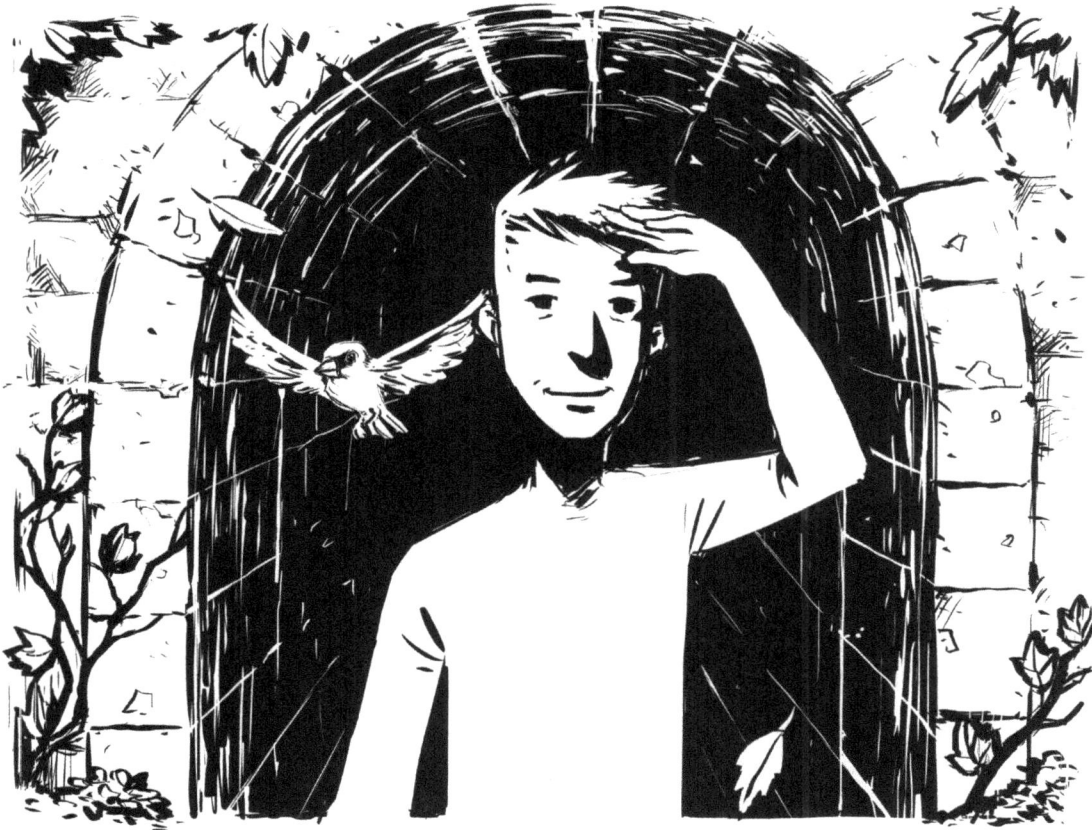

HOPE

Yes, that tiny flicker of light at the beginning of this book will get bigger and brighter over time. That is a promise, have faith.

EPILOGUE...

And always
REMEMBER...
The rain may fall, and the storm may come, but it will pass and the sun will shine again.

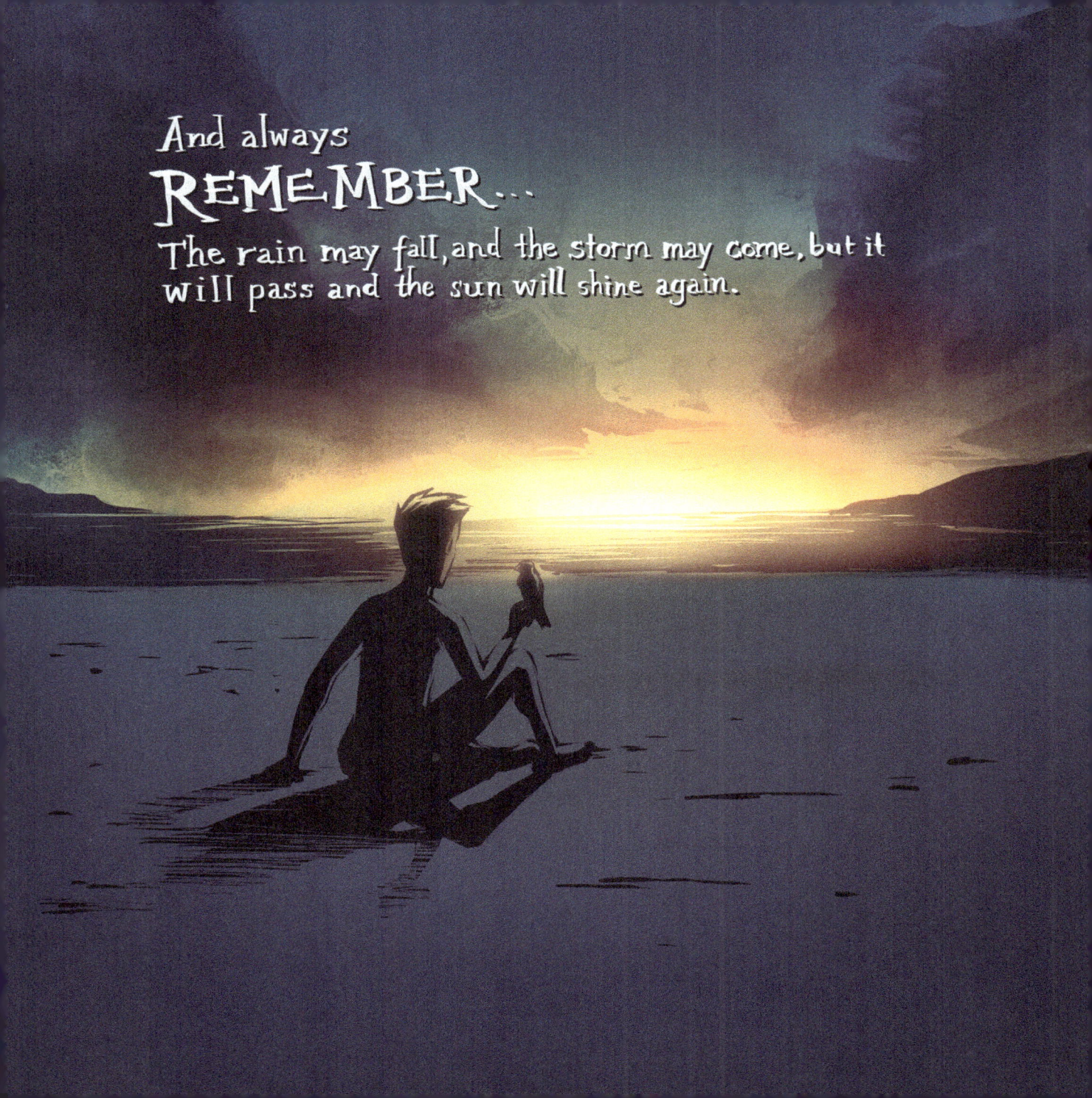

FIN.

MENTAL HEALTH TOOLKIT

CHECKLIST

Try to do at least 2 of the below every day. There maybe other activities not listed below that you enjoy or did enjoy. Keep doing them, enjoyment and satisfaction will be experienced or will return in time.

Exercise	☐	Read a book or newspaper	☑
Meditate	☐	Take a nice hot shower	☐
Socialise	☐	Go for a massage	☐
Spend time with friends	☐	Visit your favourite coffee shop	☐
Do some drawing	☐	Listen and sing along to music	☐
Take photos	☐	Do sudoku	☐
Do Yoga	☐	Play your favourite sport	☐
Cook a healthy meal	☐	Play an instrument	☐
Do some woodwork	☐	Play video games	☐
Do a jigsaw	☐	Write all the things you're grateful for	☐

GETTING HELP

Lifeline

A national charity providing all Australians experiencing a personal crisis with access to 24 hour crisis support and suicide prevention services. No one needs to face their problems alone and help is available. If you are desperate please pickup the phone and seek help from Lifeline. Call them on 13 11 14 or chat online with their crisis support team. If life is in danger CALL 000.

Beyond Blue

An independent, not-for-profit organisation supported by the Federal Government and every State and Territory Government in Australia. Striving to do everything they can to improve the lives of people affected by anxiety, depression, and suicide in Australia. Beyond Blue Support Services is available on 1300 224 636.

Your Local Doctor

A good place to start is your local GP. There is nothing to be afraid of and it's a good idea to speak with your GP if you are struggling with your mental health. Depending on the nature of the problem, your GP will conduct an assessment of you, or refer you to a mental health professional, such as a psychiatrist or a psychologist.

MEDITATION APPS

Headspace uses mindfulness and meditation to help you. The app's aim is to provide you with the essential tools to achieve a happier, healthier life. Whether you need to build healthier relationships, find a place of calm, keep your mind fit, or reduce stress, Headspace has hundreds of themed mindfulness and meditation sessions to support you.

Calm focuses on the four key areas of meditation, breathing, sleep, and relaxation, with the aim of bringing joy, clarity, and peace to your daily life. The app delivers meditations that can help you to destress, as well as breathing programs, music, and sounds from nature to relax your mind and body and promote better sleep satisfaction.

Stop, Breathe & Think promotes meditation & mindfulness to help you build the emotional strength and confidence to handle life's ups and downs. Stop, Breathe & Think allows you to check in with your emotions, and then recommends short, guided meditations, yoga and acupressure videos, tuned to how you feel.

HELPFUL BOOKS

I Had A Black Dog by Matthew Johnstone

This moving and ultimately uplifting insight into what it is like to live with Black Dog (Depression) as a companion and the strength and support that can be found within and around us to tame it. Black dog can be a terrible beast, but bringing him out of the shadows is the first steps towards recovery.

The Happiness Trap by Dr Russell Harris

How to stop struggling and start living. A user friendly guide to Acceptance Commitment Therapy (ACT). A mindfulness program for reducing stress, overcoming fear and creating a rich and meaningful life.

Self Compassion by Dr Kristin Neff

Stop Beating Yourself Up and Leave Insecurity Behind offers expert advice on how to limit self-criticism and offset its negative effects, enabling you to achieve your highest potential and a more contented, fulfilled life. This book offers exercises and action plans for dealing with every emotionally debilitating struggle.

PARTNERS

Think of 8 people that you know.

That's the number of people that die by suicide every day in Australia.

Join us in our efforts to reduce this statistic, help save lives and change the mental health landscape across Australia.

To partner with us get in touch at **caring@designtobias.com**

www.ingramcontent.com/pod-product-compliance
Lightning Source LLC
Chambersburg PA
CBHW041604260326
41914CB00012B/1386